Weight Loss

21 Delicious Breakfast Recipes To Jumpstart Your Day

Table of content

Introduction

Human progress has been marvelous, whether it is the commercial domain or the area of science and technology. But as the progress has been rapid, the change has been equally momentous. The transition brought about by different technological advancements has enabled revolutionary changes in the domains of life and health. Today, much of the daily chores for our lives which were performed by the humans themselves, are being performed by the machines.

The change in the patterns is surely enabling the humans to make the progress by leaps and bounds. The developmental changes are surely such which can never be dreamed of, without the intervention of developmental steps. But if we keep on going in one direction, it can affect the overall progress towards the destination. Same is the case with our ways of life. The involvement of machinery has made us devoid of healthful physical activity.

Weight issues have emerged as one of the most prominent trends of this evolution. Supported by the decrease in physical activity and increase in the consumption of artificial food, the human body is greatly inclined towards obesity. But the challenging world no longer allows you to entertain an unattractive body physique. The first step which you can take forward towards the weight loss is to control and monitor your diet.

These recipes will be the first step towards this venture. The recipes will be purely home based with no extra or special arrangements needed for following these recipes.

Chapter 1 – Weight Watchers- make up your Menu

In today's world everyone is busy and trapped in the challenges of a modern life style. The demanding social and professional life sometimes makes us relay ignorant about our bodily needs. No matter how much enthusiasm and vigor we may possess towards our life goals and passions, we can sustain and follow these, unless we posses a healthy and vigorous body. All the success and progress in one's life is wasteful if the body cannot sustain a healthy life pattern.

Just as the trends of living are changing, the needs and demands for sustaining healthy body are also undergoing a change. We being the generations of modern era have become so indulged in this new civilization that we cannot even look into the aftermaths of rapid advancement. The increased workloads, the decreased physical exertion and increased use of artificial and packed food are some worth mention trends which are completely destroying our health.

The increasing number of health issues being reported not only pertains to the ailments or diseases but the overall strength of the body is also an issue. One of the most prominent turned which has overwhelmed the twenty first centuries is the increased rate of obesity and weight gain.

Before we proceed towards the recipes here is an account of some guidelines for all the weight watchers who want some prominent change and results when the stand up on the weighing machines.

Eat "well"

Now it will sound scary to most of the people who want to shed several pounds within few days. But following a practical orientation I must say that shedding pounds within days is surely a trap. Do not make your body suffer from the drastic aftermaths of starving. Having a well elected diet and starving re two opposite poles. When your aim is to sustain a healthy life style and vigorous body, you cannot go for crash starving. It will ultimately result in loss of immunity and vigor.

So no matter how strange this advice may sound, but eat well. Your diet must comprise of almost all the major nutrients. No doubt you need to be conscious about fats and calories yet you cannot be totally ignorant of them

Break the monotony

If you are a weight watcher, it does not entail that you have to sustain your life upon soups and tats less boiled vegetables. One of the biggest reasons of people do not getting the obvious results for a weight loss effort is the monotony which is usually followed in the diet plan. Surely you need to be conscious about your calories but you do not need to be brutal to your body and add a pleasant and healthy assortment of dietary items in your menu.

Breakfast will drive your energy reservoir

It entails to one of the major reasons for listing the breakfast recipes. If you are conscious about your weight, it does not proclaim that you do not need a breakfast. You need a very healthy and rigorous breakfast routine. What you will eat in the morning, will devise your overall energy throughout the Day. Breakfast must be fresh, fuller and devoid of any artificial food items.

Chapter 2 – Snacks, Dip, Spreads and assorted recipes for Breakfast

1. Roasted Eggplant Dip

Ingredients:

- Eggplants – 5 Large sized
- Tahiti- 1/2 cup
- Coarse salt – ¼ teaspoon
- Lemon juice (freshly-squeezed)- 5 tablespoons
- Garlic cloves- 2 large sized
- Chili powder – ½ teaspoon
- Olive oil – 5 tablespoons
- Cumin– 1 teaspoon
- Parsley – ½ bunch
- Coriander leaves- 1/8 cup

Directions:

First of all preheat your microwave oven, about thirty minutes before, at 200 degrees Fahrenheit. Now with the help of a fork star outturning the egg plants. It will ensure the in depth cooking. Now with the hen of some knife or fork place each eggplant on the flame and cook the outermost layer of the egg plant. Keep changing the sides so that the eggplant is evenly cooked.

You can also use the gas strobe grill for this process. Now wrap these eggplants in a baking sheet and bake in ten oven for twenty minutes. Make sure that egg plant turn soft. You cause a knife for the softness check. After checking or softness let the eggplants get cool. Take out the polo. Now in blender add all the ingredients and the eggplant pulp. After getting pour from blender add the olive oil and mix well. You can use this dip for toasted pita or crackers in the breakfast.

2. **Scottish Pancakes**

Ingredients:

- Vanilla extract - 1 tablespoon
- Sea salt- ¼ teaspoon
- Honey- 2 tablespoon
- Eggs - 2 large
- Distilled water- 1 tablespoon
- Coconut oil – 5 tablespoons
- Baking powder - 5 cup
- Almond flour- 1/5 cup

Directions:

This fully enriched and healthy breakfast recipe will maintain your energy leaving you vigorous and energetic all along the day. All the mentioned ingredients, including the almond oil, honey and eggs are fully nourishing components. Splinter the eggs in a bowl and beat well along with vanilla extract, honey and water. In an additional bowl and mix the salt in the almond flour along with the baking powder combine them systematically. A better mixing will ensure fluffy dough of the flour; otherwise it will leave the lumps. Now mix the egg paste into the flour mixture. ensure that no lumps are formed and you get a uniform paste. Use a high flame skillet for heating of the oil. Start making the scoops of prepared batter in a circular motion to prepare properly sized pancakes. Bake each of the side for a minimum of five minutes.

3. Mushroom Pita delight

Ingredients:

- ➤ Turkey patties (crumbled) - ¼ cup
- ➤ Salt- ½ tablespoon
- ➤ Pepper – 1 tablespoon
- ➤ Paprika powder- 1/5 tablespoon
- ➤ Onions (roughly chopped)- 2 medium sized
- ➤ Mushrooms- 5 (sliced)
- ➤ Garlic powder- ½ teaspoon
- ➤ Eggs – 5 medium sized
- ➤ Dried thyme- ½ teaspoon

Directions:

The accurate whipping of the eggs is the most crucial part of this recipe, so as long as the eggs are beaten in an even manner, preparations will be done well. When you thoroughly whip the eggs start mixing all the other ingredients in this beaten mixture. Addition of other ingredients will turn this frothy mixture into a thick paste like material. But the formation of lumps is not a good sign. It will hinder efficient cooking. Once a devoid of any lumps, this paste will be then poured in to the dish. A Pyrex dish is the most suitable one. Set the mixture aside for five minutes and in the interim preheat your microwave oven at a temperature of about 200 degrees Fahrenheit. Place the tray in the oven and bake for a duration of thirty minutes.

3. **Thriving green Omlete**

Ingredients:

- Salt – 1 pinch
- Minced chicken – 50 oz
- Eggs- 2 medium sized
- Cayenne pepper – 2 tablespoons
- Butter- 2 teaspoons
- Baby spinach (finely chopped)—1 cup
- Thyme- 2 teaspoons
- Parsley- 1 cup

Directions:

Rest a cooking pan over low heat and thaw butter over low heat. When it starts giving the bubbles, mix the rinsed chicken and let it fry for five additional minutes on the same low flame. When you will notice the change in color of the chicken, from pinkish to golden brown, it is the appropriate time to mix the pepper along with the salt. In an additional bowl whisk the eggs with the remaining ingredients and little by little pour over the fried chicken. Each side of the omlete must be thoroughly cooked. It will take around three minutes for each of the side. Now garnish with the mentioned quantity of thyme and parsley.

4. Coconut filled Porridge

Ingredients:

- Coconut milk- 1/2 cup
- Almond flour- 1 cup
- Flaxseed- 2 tablespoon
- Honey – 3 tablespoons
- Salt- 1 teaspoon
- Shredded coconut (unsweetened)— 1 cup
- Vanilla essence- 1 tablespoon

Directions:

This porridge is extremely abundant in the utilities of natural coconut, so your morning will glitter and glisten with this brisk and dynamic breakfast. Eating coconut in the morning provides the additional benefits of calcium and benefits. First of all heat the coconut milk till it simmers three to four times. Vanilla essence will be added in the boiled milk. Keep stirring after addition of the essence. Mix the remaining ingredients one after the other. Cook on low intensity flame. It will need around fifteen minutes. Serve with shredded almonds.

5. Kale With Green Eggs

Ingredients:

- Sea salt – 1/2 teaspoon
- Kale leaves- 6
- Eggs- 4 large sized
- Coconut oil- ½ cup
- Chicken loaf - 4 slices
-

Directions:

Whisk the eggs gently. Now tale the electric blender and the kale leave along with the whisked eggs. Add the salt. Blend the mixture for almost five minutes. Set aside, this thick mixture. Now heat up a saucepan with oil and insert the chicken loaf to get fired from each of the two sides. In the additional pan place the whisked egg and cook like an omlete. These two mixtures will be baked together over the iron skillet.

6. Luscious banquet Bars

Ingredients:

- ➤ Vanilla extract- 1teaspoon
- ➤ Sea salt – ¼ teaspoon
- ➤ Raisins- 1/8 cup
- ➤ Pumpkin seeds- ¼ cup
- ➤ One fourth cup of sunflower seeds - ½ cup
- ➤ Honey- 2 tablespoon
- ➤ Distilled water- 2 tablespoon
- ➤ Coconut shreds(unsweetened)- ½ cup
- ➤ Coconut oil- 2 tablespoon
- ➤ Almonds (sliced) - ½ cup
- ➤ Almond flour (pale)- half cup

Directions:

You will need an electric food processor to carefully mix flour and the salt. Mix oil and vanilla essence, one by one. Keep the mixture aside. In a blender mix all the seeds and the shredded coconut. Blend fine for five minutes. Now put the mixtures to form dough like stuff. Use a 10x15 Pyrex dish to put the mixture. You can also use knife for forming large bars of the dough. Now cook it for about ten minutes at a temperature of 250 degrees Fahrenheit. Serve refrigerated.

7. Banana filled Breakfast Cookies for weight watchers

Ingredients:

- Strawberry (chopped)- 2 tablespoons
- whole dates – 5
- Shredded coconut (unsweetened)- 1/2 cup
- Sea salt- 1 teaspoon
- Raisins- ½ cup
- Pecans (chopped) - 2 tablespoons
- Nutmeg – 1 teaspoon
- Eggs - 3
- Coconut flour - 1 cup
- Cinnamon – 1 teaspoon
- Bananas - 3 medium sized
- Baking powder– 1 teaspoon
- Almond butter - 1 cup
- Vanilla essence – 1 teaspoon

Directions:

Steep the dates in high warm water. It will give you the pitted dates. Use the food processor to mix the almond butter, coconut flour and date. Add the well enthused eggs, vanilla essence cinnamon, salt, shredded coconut and baking powder. Mix all of these ingredients again.

Now make small scoops of this dough. You will add the nuts and the raisins with an intention to make the dough more nourishing and healthy. Dip in the egg mixture and fry in the oil.

8. Light Porridge

Ingredients:

- Vanilla essence – 2 teaspoon
- Sea salt – 1 teaspoon
- Raw honey – 3 teaspoons
- Milk (Cold)- 1 litre
- Eggs– 3
- Crushed pecans – 1/2 cup
- Coconut (Unsweetened)– 1 cup
- Cinnamon (powdered) – 1/2 teaspoon

Directions:

Immerse the frayed coconut in the chilled milk for about two hours before the preparation of the recipe. Now put the cooking bowl over a low intensity flame and cook the mixture until milk gets into the coconut pieces and only half of the original amount is left. Put off the flame and add the other ingredients into the combination. Blend it well. Utilize a casserole large dish for cooking. Cook for at least fifteen minute at a temperature of about 250 degrees Fahrenheit.

9. Breakfast Muffins

Ingredients:

- ➢ Strawberries- 10 whole
- ➢ Ground flax – 1 tablespoon
- ➢ Dates- 5 large sized
- ➢ Coconut milk – ¼ cup
- ➢ Bananas- 2 large sized
- ➢ Almond meal- ½ cup

Directions:

First of all you need make a thick paste of the strawberries. Make a thick puree and leave it aside. In an additional bowl start putting the ground flax, dates and the almond meal. Put in the blender to ensure that it turn out to be a paste. Now pour the oil and the coconut milk into the blended mixture. Place the mixture on a large muffin tray and start placing the strawberry topping on each piece of the muffin. When developed place the muffins in refrigerator to get solidified and chilled. Thaw twenty minutes prior to consumption.

10. Carrot and coconut breakfast Recipe

Ingredients:

- Spinach – 1 cup
- Salt- 2 teaspoons
- pepper– 1 teaspoon
- garlic (Minced)– 2 teaspoon
- Leeks (sliced) – 1/2 cup
- Eggs - 2
- Coconut oil – 4 teaspoons
- Carrots (thinly sliced) – 1 cup

Directions:

Heat the coconut oil on aflame of low intensity and use it for frying the leeks, the garlic, and the carrots. It will take around fifteen minutes. Now put in spinach and continue stirring constantly. Awaiting the vegetables to turn crispy, keep frying. Now turn off the flame. In an additional bowl, blend the eggs with pepper and salt. Fry this mixture to prepare omlete. Now cover the omlete in a dish and pour the fried vegetables evenly. Serve hot.

11. Breakfast in Burrito style

Ingredients:

- Ham (sliced)- 2 per serving
- Olive oil- 4 tablespoons
- Mix vegetables as per the availability– 2 cups
- Eggs – 3

Directions:

Stir fry all the selected vegetables for about eight minutes in the arranged quantity of the olive oil. Beat the egg in a large bowl and pour over the vegetables. Bake it thoroughly until the egg gets golden brown. In a separate pan deep fry the ham. Make sure it is cooked from both sides. In a medium plate place ham and cover with burrito. Sprinkle the salad sauce according to the taste.

12. Spring Casseroles

Ingredients:

- ➢ Tomatoes (diced) – ½ cup
- ➢ Sweet potato (sliced) – ½ cup
- ➢ Sausage – 2 cups
- ➢ Salt – 2 teaspoons
- ➢ Pepper – 2 teaspoons
- ➢ Green onion – 2 small sizes
- ➢ Egg– 1
- ➢ Baby spinach (thoroughly chopped) – 1 cup

Directions:

USE a non stick pan for cooking the sausage. It will take around four to five minutes. Use a large pan for frying the vegetables. You will start with onion and sweet potatoes and spinach will be added at the end. It will take ten minutes. When fried pour the sausage and mix gently. In a baking dish pour some melted butter. Now make layers of the two mixtures one over the other. Now beat the eggs and add the pepper and salt. Pour the egg mixture over the tray. Now take a preheated microwave oven to cook the rolls at about 400 degrees Fahrenheit and for duration of 20 minutes. When baking is done, get a sharp knife and cut serving squares.

13. Fruit lover's Breakfast

Ingredients:

- kiwis (peeled) – 3 large sized
- Pineapple slices – 2 cups
- Organic Honey – 3 tablespoon
- Green grapes- 1 cup
- lemon juice (Fresh)- 3 tablespoons
- Blueberries- 4 whole
- Apples (diced) – 2 large sized

Directions:

First of all for hygienic surety thoroughly rinse all the fresh fruits. Make sure you get to the fresh fruits, rather than packed or tinned. Now cut them into a fine size which looks good upon serving. Add in a serving bowl and mix all the ingredients. The drizzling lemon juice will give extra benefits to the weight watchers. This fruity breakfast will maintain your energy reservoirs full all along the day long without much anxiety of calorie gain.

14. Shrimp Avocado Omlete

Ingredients:

- ➢ Tomato (chopped) – 3 whole
- ➢ Shrimp (peeled) – 2 lb
- ➢ Olive oil – 1 cup
- ➢ Eggs- 3 large sized
- ➢ Avocado (assorted) – 1 large size

Directions:

Carefully rinse the shrimps under the running water. Let the eat dry under air. Now shift in a pan with oil, to sauté well. When the shrimps starts giving pinkish look, it is a signal that it is well cooked. Now prepare a bowl for whipping the eggs and also mix the avocado and onions. Beat it well and decant in the pan. Bake until the egg give golden brown look. In the meantime cut the prepared shrimps in even pieces. When the egg is cooked, extend the shrimp mixture on the egg, leaving half side as empty. Now use the other empty half of the egg for making the wrap.

15. Delectable Pumpkin Pancakes

Ingredients:

- Sea salt – 1/4 teaspoon
- Pumpkin spices– 2 teaspoons
- Pumpkin puree- 2 cups
- Maple syrup – 1/2 teaspoon
- Flax seeds– 1/ 4 cup
- Eggs- 3 small
- Cinnamon (powdered)– 2 teaspoon
- Butter- 100 oz
- Baking soda- 2 tablespoons
- Apple cider vinegar – 2 teaspoons
- Almond milk – 1 cup
- Almond flour (lightened) – 2 cups

Directions:

Whip the gees gently. No take a bowl to mix thoroughly the almond flour and the beaten eggs. Blend them with a wire whisk or electric beater if not formed into a consistent uniform firm mixture. In this mixture start adding the pumpkin puree. Continuous stirring is needed while mixing every ingredient. It will ensure that not any of the ingredients comes out in the form of the lump. Mix baking soda when you are done with the puree. Adding it earlier will make the mixture fluffier. Add butter in the non stock pan and keep the flame on low. With a large size spoon begin adding the prepared batter. Turn over the sides of the batter frequently, to stay away from the unprepared lumps.

16. Eggplant breakfast

Ingredients:

- ➢ Salt – a pinch
- ➢ Pepper- 2 teaspoon
- ➢ Olive oil- 4 cup
- ➢ Eggs- 3 medium sized
- ➢ Eggplants (thinly cut in the shape of discs)- 3 large

Directions:

Preheat the skillet very carefully for this recipe. Pour the olive oil on to the cooking skillet. Thoroughly beat the eggs with an electric beater. When it gives out white frothy appearance add the salt and the pepper and mix with a spoon. Try to keep it fluffy. Adding some drops of water while beating the eggs will make certain that the eggs come out to be fluffier. Now start dipping the finely cut eggplant disc into the beaten egg mixture. Leave for few seconds in the mixture. You can either use a skillet or you can even sauté these discs in a non stick frying pan.

17. Coconut Waffles

Ingredients:

- Vanilla extract- 2 teaspoon
- Honey- 4 tablespoons
- Eggs- 2 small sized
- Coconut sugar- 1/4 cup
- Coconut oil- 1/4 cup
- Coconut milk – 4 tablespoon
- Baking soda- 1/6 tablespoon
- Almond flour- 2 cups

Directions:

The success of this recipe lies in the way you make the dough for it. The dough must be consistent and all the ingredients must be thoroughly mixed. Start making the dough and make a mixture of baking soda and almond flour. When you are sure that ingredients are well mixed, start pouring the milk slowly. Do not over spill. In the end add the vanilla extract and mix again. You will need a waffle iron to bake the waffles. Start pouring the dough mixture over the almond waffles. Now take two large pots. One will be filled with coconut oil and the other will be containing the coconut sugar. When you are sure that they are thoroughly cooked. Dip each of it in the coconut oil and coconut sugar successively. Leave the waffle dipped for few second in each ingredient. It will ensure that a thick coating is formed over the surface of the waffle. You can also sprinkle chopped coconut over the waffles

18. Prosciutto Cups

Ingredients:

- Prosciutto – 1 slice
- Pepper – up to taste
- Egg – 2 large sized
- Vinegar- 1 tablespoon
- Basil leaves- 1 teaspoon

Directions:

First of all heat the Prosciutto slices over a grill. You can either use a cooking oven or an iron skillet. In this recipe you need to make preparations for your microwave oven. Take a parchment paper and keep it for lining the tin for the cooking of the Prosciutto. Now brush the slices with olive oil. Does not use more than a few drop. Now keep these slices as a lining for the baking tin. Make this lining very evenly; otherwise the cooking will not be thorough. The base and vertical sides of the tin need to be evenly enclosed with Prosciutto slices. Use the same tin for enabling other ingredients to be the part of slices. Now over this used tin make a layer of the eggs and sprinkle the pepper according to your taste inclination. After preparing give it few minutes to settle, most probably, ten minutes. Now keep the prepared baking tin in the microwave oven and bake for about 30 minutes, at a temperature of about 250 degrees Fahrenheit.

19. Vegetable twist in Scrambled Eggs with veggie twist

Ingredients:

- ➢ Tomatoes (sliced)- 2 whole
- ➢ Spring onions (chopped) – 2 large size
- ➢ Mushrooms- 1 cup
- ➢ Eggs - 5
- ➢ Cubed ham- 1 cup
- ➢ Vegetable oil- 1 teaspoon
- ➢ Parsley (chopped) – ¼ cup

Directions:

You can use any of the available cooking oil or the making of this recipe, but if you are a weight watcher then I will suggest you to preferably use olive oil. This oil is especially helpful if you do not want a calorie gain you need to get hold of the olive oil. Now take a small quantity of oil in a large size pan. Large pan will ensure thorough cooking. Fry the tomatoes and onions, one by one. After that you need to fry the mushrooms. Over fried mushrooms will eventually cause a loss of real flavour which is the characteristic of mushrooms. Now make the preparations for the omlete. For that whisk the eggs and add the pepper and salt. Make a yellowish golden egg and set aside. Mash the fried omlete into small pieces with the help of the fork. Now spread the scrambled egg over a serving dish. Then put over the hem and garnish with fried tomatoes and onions. Sprinkle the chopped parsley evenly.

20.   Ham Salad with Hardboiled Eggs and veggies

Ingredients:

- Tomato (evenly sliced) - 1
- Spinach (finely chopped) – 1 cup
- Soya sauce- 3 teaspoons
- Ham – 10 slices
- Green onion – 2 medium
- Eggs - 4
- Coconut oil – 2 tablespoon
- Celery chopped- 2 fresh stalks
- Carrot – 1 whole
- Broccoli (sliced)- 1
- Avocado (chopped) – 1 large

Directions:

First of all take water in a large bowl. Add a pinch of salt in this water. We will be using this water for boiling the eggs. Cover the pan with a lid. When you think that the eggs are done, immediately shift the eggs under the running water. It will aid in easy peeling off the egg shell. Do not keep the eggs half boiled, for that you may need to boil for five to eight minutes. Gently peel off the shell of the eggs. Now cut the eggs into evenly sized and thin discs. Now rinse all the vegetables one by one and cut into the shape which is prescribed in the ingredients chart. Stir fry these vegetables in a small quantity of coconut oil. Now rinse the ham slices and use an iron skillet for cooking the ham. Mix all the assorted vegetables to make a dressing without oil. In a serving dish make a layer of vegetables and then keep a ham slice e over it. Now make a layer of egg discs. Cover it with another hem slice. Pour the soya sauce and serve hot. You can alternatively use apple cider vinegar for accounting the weight issues.

21. Salmon Patties for weight watchers

Ingredients:

- Vinegar – 1 tablespoon
- Scallions (chopped)- ¼ cup
- Salmon (skin removed)- 1 lb
- Minced garlic – 1 tablespoon
- Fresh ginger (mashed) – 1 tablespoon
- Eggs – 2 large size
- Coconut oil– 2 tablespoons
- Coconut flour – 1 tablespoon
- Parsley- ½ cup

Directions:

First of all rinse thoroughly the salmon and leave it to get dry for almost fifteen minutes under the fan or in the pleasant air. When it gets dried out, incise into tiny cubes. The accurate cutting of salmon is very critical for effective and though cooking. The precise sized cubes will make sure a deep cooking. Now take a medium sized bowl and beat the eggs. Whip all the eggs rigorously. The frothy egg whips will allow an effective inclusion into the meat. Add the ginger and garlic according to the prescribed quantity. Leave it for few minutes. Now prepare your iron skillet. Clean ait thoroughly and brush it prescribed amount of coconut oil. Now burn the flame and keep the intensity very much low. Now pour the finely cut salmon cubes in the whisked egg mixture. In a separate bowl take the coconut flour and use it for dipping the dip the salmon cubes, after dipping into the egg mixture. Put over the heated skillet one by one. Gently cook both sides of the meat but ensure that it is not over cooked.

Conclusion

The human life trends have changed dramatically. The extensive physical activity which was once a part of human civilization has greatly reduced. Today the energy driven physical burdens have been over taken by the sophisticated machines. As a result there has been a rapid decrease in the physical activity in the daily household. Not only the physical activity has been cut short but the there has been vast change in the eating patterns of today's human civilization. These eating patterns are usually governed by the artificial food additives and processed edibles.

But how has this change impacted the human civilization as a whole. The aftermaths have been both positive as well as negative. On the brighter side these have cut across all the limits of progress and utility and on the dark corners you can see the negative effects in the form of increased health concerns and body ailments. One such effect which is largely being reported in different parts of the world includes the weight gain problem ultimately leading to obesity and plumpness. But nobody wants it.

These recipes are a special gift for all the weight watchers who want to enjoy the flavors of food without disturbing the body pounds. The collection specially pertains to the breakfast recipes which can make your day. A good breakfast at the beginning of the day will clearly set your pace for an energetic day. The recipes provide a wide assortment of taste and ingredients so that you may not get fed up of one type of food being consumed all the day.